Conversations about Hypnosis and other Mind Stuff

Insights into the World of Hypnosis with Ines Simpson

Taken from Ines's Podcasts on Hypnosis-Everywhere and a series of Articles originally posted on LinkedIn. The articles are in dialogue form to give the back and forth insights into the different aspects of Hypnosis. And the Fact and Fallacies that surround the word and the world of Hypnosis.

Cover Photo by Tanja Heffner on Unsplash

Table of Contents

Hi my name is Ines Simpson and I want to introduce you to my World of Hypnosis

It's a lot like your world — but with benefits!!

The Hypnotist, I find tends to live in a world of Belief and Forgiveness, as opposed to a world of Fact, Truth and Blame

The Hypnotist is also dealing with the mind, a slippery creature that just when you think you have figured it out — its shows a new color

Some colors can be very dark sometimes, but when they are removed, painlessly by the way, and this is my job after all, to remove the dark places from your mind, when you take them away and reveal the rest — it's a brilliant , colorful place to work in

So welcome, explore and investigate my world.

Ines

Ines Simpson - Who is she?

(also see bio at end)

Ines Simpson is an Internationally Awarded Hypnotist and Hypnosis Trainer

- Won the 2012 Hallmark award at the NGH convention (best instructor as voted by attendees).
- Board Certified instructor for National Guild of Hypnotists.
- Became a Member of the Braid – National Guild of Hypnotists.
- Certified Hypnotherapist – International Medical & Dental Hypnotherapy Association.
- Certified Instructor for Omni Hypnosis Training
- Won award for "HYPNOSIS PIONEER" in Zurich. Switzerland for her development of Simpson Protocol (SP) Advanced Hypnosis.
- Development Of "Simpson Protocol" started over a decade ago and continues to evolve   and expand.
- She teaches Hypnosis and Advanced Hypnosis Courses in Canada ,USA, S. America, Europe, Dubai.

Hypnosis

as a natural event
as a concept
as a career
a profession
part time income
a hobby
a life of helping others
and most importantly
as your very own self-help course
that works!

"Hypnosis is nothing but a vehicle or gateway to allow us to connect to the best and ultimate parts of us. It's still us. It's just the BEST PART of us." *Ines Simpson*

All Hypnosis is Self -Hypnosis

No-one hypnotizes another, the person being hypnotized must allow themselves to fall into a hypnotic state. A state they can emerge from at any time, at will.

The hypnotist only achieves their outcomes if the client ultimately trusts the hypnotists. If here is no connection the hypnosis will have no effect. The hypnotist merely guides and facilitates. The client allows his or her own mind to do its work.

'official ' definition
On March 24th, 2014, the APA (American Psychological Association) has accepted the following definitions:

Hypnosis: *"a state of consciousness involving focused attention and reduced peripheral awareness characterized by an enhanced capacity for response to suggestions."*

Hypnotic induction: *"a procedure designed to induce hypnosis."*

Hypnotherapy:*"the use of hypnosis in the treatment of a medical or psychological disorder or concern."*

We could say going into a hypnotic state is merely a way of saying you change states from Distracted to Focused.

We could say in fact Hypnosis, in its broadest sense – is the Language of the Mind

PART ONE

Hypnosis is everywhere?

To answer that question – yes Hypnosis is everywhere – all the time. It is as much an essential of humanity as breathing, heart beat and blood flow. Hypnosis is the language of the mind.

Take the broad spectrum definition of Hypnosis : Hypnosis occurs or is occurring when there is a change of mental state and focus becomes concentrated to the exclusion of everyday learned logic.

This what happens when we watch an enjoyable movie that engross us, or read a book, or are 'captivated' by another human, because of their looks, or charisma, or attitude or energy.

This what is happening when commercials through images or word association are watched by you.

Or speeches by leaders who demand our attention and admiration by words and actions placed and used by deliberation or talent.

This is what happens in sports when the participant visualizes the play, the swing , the stroke.
This is what is happening when the sergeant major yells and the new recruits – happens to both parties.

This is what happens in trauma , or when we walk into a hospital – or go back to our parents and become the 30 years old child. We change states of mind. By-pass the critical factor of our everyday logic (I am 30 years old not a child)

This is what is happens when we are daydreaming at work or in a class.

This is what is happening when we are engrossed in the work or class

Hypnosis is happening all the time to all of us – and it passes through us the same way air passes through our lungs – naturally.

And like breathing sometimes , unintentionally, and without awareness we allow in 'bad' hypnosis., as we sometimes breathe in bad air.

When we are not told that we are being led into a light hypnotic state – Advertising for instance, car ads, beer ads, lifestyle ads – where the pictures show attractive images that have nothing to with the product but suggest those dreams can be yours if you buy the product.
Or where Leadership uses words that conjure up images that are only there to suggest things never said.
They are setting triggers and compounding suggestions, that you are only half aware of.
Light hypnosis done without permission.

So yes Hypnosis is everywhere. Be aware.

But then there is the tighter more formal acceptance of hypnosis – formal hypnosis where either on a stage with carefully hand picked volunteers or in an office with a client who is ready to change.

Formal Hypnosis where the Hypnotists leads the client or volunteers into hypnosis, hypnosis all parties desire and accept – and can refuse at any step of the way.

Hypnosis is always a choice.

You can choose to daydream or be enthralled or you can snap out of it – by choice. Just as you can choose to hold your breath or not, at any time.

You can choose Hypnosis to change your state and life for the better.

You can choose to allow that 'inner' mind to guide you, learn how, or not.

Free will states that our Inner or Higher mind will never override our conscious will, even though our will is quite weak.

So it's a choice. Our life is a result of choices we make.

And the more we understand the power of our mind - the better our choices.

Where did Hypnosis come from?

It came from and comes from the natural interaction of our minds with that we call reality. Conscious and Subconscious interacting.

Asking where it came from, in the end , is asking where breathing came from – it's part of us (see Hypnosis Everywhere)

But if we ask where did the formal practice of Modern Hypnotherapy (that is Hypnosis used deliberately to relieve stress, anxiety and pain etc.) then it comes directly from the medical community in the 18th and 19th century.

It comes from a time when the Mind Body connection was considering important to healing. As technology and drugs moved into the medical arena – there was a change in direction of medicine from the concept of healing holistically to healing symptoms.

Medicine in the 19th and 20th century moved into the Industrial technological age where you break things down to their component parts and then work on the components. Whether that is conveyor belt manufacturing or 'fixing' a symptom.

As technology became more expensive and a must-have for hospitals – the best MRI machines, the CAT Scan technology – the administrations clamoring to have the latest state- of the -art tech ,so they can put them in their prospectus. Costs escalated. As costs escalated more and more patients had to be run through the machinery for best cost benefit ratios. Doctors have 7 minutes to work with a patient, Surgeons are tired, overworked, and stressed .

Suicide is at an all-time high in the Medical Community.

The person, the individual disappears from medicine.

As Big Pharma realized the wealth in creating 'illnesses' and then supplying drugs for them – the reason for healing disappeared and the power of money makes it appear that there is a need to maintaining constant illness.

Add in the Insurance companies cut and you can see why Health Care is staggeringly expensive – so many hands are taking, and have a vested interest in keeping costs and profits high. (see Turing Pharmaceuticals fraud case with Martin Shkreli as one example – and the manufactured Opioid crisis as another- report here- https://www.theguardian.com/us-news/2017/oct/19/big-pharma-money-lobbying-us-opioid-crisis).

However as Hospitals stagger under their own costs – anything that can bring costs down is now welcomed. And so we see Hypnosis coming back.

It is used and being taught in Trauma Wards where when Hypnosis is used there are less drugs used (less cost) , doctors work with patients who are not stressed, and who are primed to heal. Thus there is quicker turnaround time and much faster (natural) healing.

Hypnosis is being used again surgery – again faster operation time and faster healing – freeing up beds.

Hypnosis is used in Pain centers – less opioid use and therefore less long term cost to the system

Hypnosis is used in the Mayo Clinic and hospitals in Belgium.

Patients arrive less stressed, easier to work with and faster healing time as the body is allowed to work without the stultifying load of being drugged.

However Hypnosis is still not taught in medical schools – except maybe one day of 'Progressive Relaxation techniques and Direct

Suggestion – which is old style hypnosis. Useful, but hardly a complete course.

The average doctor has maybe 6 hours 'training' in Hypnosis, whereas the average Stage Hypnotist, never mind Hypnotherapist, will have hundreds of hours of training.

And yet Dave Elman, in the 1950's taught exclusively doctors, dentists and psychiatrists to use 60 second inductions and 5 to 10 minute sessions to relive pain, anxiety , what we would now call PTYSD etc.

But so now the biggest benefit to the health care system hypnosis offers is that anyone can learn it – its short term fast therapy and is extremely effective and cheap.

Hypnosis treats the whole person - mind body and spirit and allows the body and mind to do what they do best – heal and repair.

Hypnosis de-stresses and gives back control for healing to the individual.

But the biggest downside as far as corporations and doctors have – is how to monetize a natural occurring process.

Then there is also the challenge that with hypnosis the body actually heals – and there is less and less repeat business from individual patients.

This goes against the apparent current Medical industry's mantra of ' create a symptom, make a drug'.   As someone once said the Medical Industry is, by its nature, in the business of illness not health.

Hypnosis allows the individual to remove dis-ease and take back control of their healing.

We are always going to need doctors and surgeons and nurses and hospitals.

But perhaps they will go back to treating the whole person ,
removing disease from individuals and giving them back their whole
body. Not just pieces of it.

Hypnosis controls you doesn't it

Is Hypnosis really something I choose?

All hypnosis is self-hypnosis. That is no-one 'hypnotizes' you. You accept the hypnosis. You accept the images the ads flash at you (without your permission note) you listen to the leaders speeches because they tell you, your friends tell you – your boss tells you.

But that's a choice. You allow the stage hypnotist to lead you into hypnosis – because you want to have fun and you want to play.

And you choose to allow the Hypnotist to lead you into hypnosis because you want the anxiety or phobia or habit to be once and for all – gone. It's a choice

But you say- what about hypnosis and control – what about let's say brain washing – isn't that real?.

If it wasn't then there have been billions of dollars spent by Proctor and Gamble and Budweiser and Gm that have gone to waste!!

Brain washing – say in a prison environment or coercive situation – even say the military for its recruits – it takes a lot of breaking of the 'will' and then building back up with suggestion and compounded (many times given) suggestion. It takes a long time.

You don't buy Tide because of one commercial – it is because of repetition and peer pressure and compounded suggestion. Light brain washing our society does all the time.

So then the Hypnotizer has control?

No in those situations we give up – by choice (because we are beaten or tired or overwhelmed or deliberately confused for a long time. And we give up.

Just as a leader knows if you tell the big lie and keep telling it over and over – eventually the listener becomes overwhelmed and confused and can no longer remember how to judge truth or fiction.

So any leader who abuses his position as one who by the nature of his position exudes authority (light hypnosis again) and uses that position to confuse and deride – is often believed because of the weight of the fiction and lies and because there is no counter weight.

He has authority and by our natures we give authority the benefit of the doubt. We allow our critical factor to be over ridden (a definition of hypnosis)

But also it is a choice by us not to step back and analyze.

The Stage Hypnotist, the Hypnotherapist – in their one or two hour sessions have no hope of 'controlling' or brain washing. They only want you to choose to allow the benefits.

The Stage Hypnotist the advantage though of peer pressure from an audience and the luxury of choosing the 5 or 10 volunteers who will allow the most.

The Hypnotherapist only deals with people who want the best outcomes and are prepared to make the one or two hour mind journey to get that outcome

So yes Hypnosis is everywhere and happening all the time – and is as necessary to our mind as breathing is to our physical system.

And we choose the benefits. Or choose to ignore the obvious call to be 'hypnotized' by the leader on the podium or the corporation with its shrill demands to buy.

All Hypnosis is not Equal

(spoiler alert – could be a rant!!)

Taking the broad inclusive definition of Hypnosis – that is a change of state where focus becomes either intense or distracted – and thus messages not normally accepted readily can be accepted without the normal filters – then, in a world such as ours there are many ready to take advantage of that.

Detrimental or Manipulative Hypnosis then.

Possibly you immediately think of the Stage Hypnotists making spectacles of the volunteers, or perhaps the Stage Magician where distraction and misdirection are everything (well everything, let's not forget the endless hours of practice, and the hundreds of dollars spent on the 'magical' equipment).

But these professions are non-descript, minor, in their negative effect on us – compared to the main users of Hypnosis for manipulation in our societies.

There is, for example, the advertising community – who spend thousands, millions, of dollars and years of research to manipulate their target audience – us. Research on waking hypnosis that is - which visual stimuli, sound, color, and yes smell create by-pass. Anything to by-pass distract or misdirect to get that message past our critical factor.

In grocery stores endless research is undergone to search out where our triggers are. What creates this mood or that? What color, what music, what word? Triggers that move us to pick this or that brand. Where are eyes travel when we look at shelves, which colors are attractive, which colors evoke trust, which colors evoke action to buy.

Where to place Dairy and where to place Bread.

Which items work best at the cash counter, on the end of the aisle, and which end of aisles work better than others.

All boxes and cans and bottles and jars are not just randomly selected – and their labels are not just there because they are pretty – or reflect a designer's flourishing art career.

A Major Grocery Store is the battleground for your mind and eye. Competing brands use multi strategies to claim your attention – then provoke an action. It's all suggestion, compounded suggestions and misdirection directed at you, at us. Intentionally, deliberately and with only one desire -to make you buy.

Food companies spend millions of dollars on what word triggers a reaction to their product – 'organic' 'fresh', 'gluten free', 'Healthy', 'no sugar added', 'sugar free', 'diet', 'green', 'healthy', 'simple', 'no chemicals added', 'vegan safe' Etc. etc. None of these words on food products are saying what you think they are saying. But they are selected for you deliberately – just as a stage hypnotist selects his or her volunteers – carefully.
Hypnosis always works.

But then so what we might say? It's not stealing – we need to buy food anyway. However, we are led in most cases by misdirection and the compounding of suggestion to which brand or bottle or label we buy.

Those FRESH vegetables in those country farm looking barrels and boxes – have traveled hundreds of miles and been dowsed with who knows how many chemicals so that they arrive weeks later in that store looking ripe and colorful and 'fresh' An illusion of chemicals and technical expertise, and our willingness to suspend disbelief.

The drug companies – despite their mile a minute waiver at the end of ads – tell us what we want to hear. This dug creates calm, this drug sleep, this an erection. And when they run out of things they make 'dis-ease' up to fit the drug. IBS, ADD, RLS, PTSD.

Now yes, we have bowel problems and some, few, very few, and hyper active kids. However as we know, anxiety and stress are pretty much rampant.

But none of these are dis-eases.

Even though we know and they know its blatant deceptive advertising. But they know we will always hope – that this or that drug will cure what ails us. We will allow our critical factor to be by-passed by stories and calculated emotional messages happen.

Many television or video ads have the budget of a movie. And the editing is even more carefully applied than a big budget movie – because they need to convey 'the message' in a few minutes or even a few seconds. And because we fast forward the ads, or mute them, they have to convey the message in a few visuals – and they do. They don't do all that research for nothing. Hypnosis is possibly the most researched profession in the advertising world.

Now even a 12-year-old now learns how to craft their YouTube vide for maximum 'clicks'.

It's our minds they are seeking to attract. Our attention.

And there is only one way to do that without force and that is through Hypnosis. By passing the normal protective filters we may have up and getting the message into our psyche.

And now the noise about the 'fake news' episodes – attracting targeted people to act in ways they wouldn't act without the fake news message. Stealing profiles from your Facebook, Twitter, Snapchat profile to manipulate you more. An inside job!

However, all 'news' shows are biased to a targeted audience.

Nowhere does a network or organization don't randomly spew 'news at you. All news programs are vehicles for advertising and or agendas.

And it's not necessarily always clear what that might be.

When you volunteer to go on stage with a stage hypnotist – you are pretty aware of what you are doing.

Advertisers offer no clear parameters -they only have one overarching desire – to grab your attention – whether you volunteer or not-and then take your, our money.

Politicians hire speech writers and pollsters not because they are unable to speak – but because they know they just can't say what they mean - they need their agenda to be carried through the 'noise' that surrounds us and them. So catch phrases, simple promises and words that call for action, or fear, or hate are the easiest crowd pleasers. They do not presume to be talking casually to someone in a coffee shop. They are trying to raise the energy to action of thousands of people. They are working to and for the mob mentality.

Pharmaceutical companies don't market a drug – they market a narrative – the story of what it will do for you, for us. And yet, as the companies themselves well know – the drug of choice of Americans – the 'anti-depressant '– they have no real idea of how or why it works. As Lauren Slater says in her book 'Blue Dreams' – when we take the drug – are we taking the drug or the story that comes with it? Both seem to have side effects.

Cosmetic companies sell the smell, the feel, the glamour – the feel of the lotion, the smell of the perfume hypnotize us into believing results and consequences that have no bearing on the minerals and chemicals that are actually in the potions.

Casinos spends inordinate amounts of money on manipulating us to stay gambling in their casinos. Of course, we contribute by allowing ourselves to be hypnotized by the lure of the big win or the fun in the casino, lady luck, lucky hands, unlucky hands, lucky colors unlucky colors.

But a simple thing like the slot machine, the one-armed bandit (rightly named) is a huge money maker for the casino and they have spent years and millions of research dollar on how to precisely and exactly make those lights flash just right and the sounds to ring out just right – so that they (literally) induce a trance. A person no longer cares win or lose – they just want to stay there in that safe place with their machine and its friendly lights and sounds – away from the worries of the world. Complete trance is their objective. The Zen state of gambling.

And crowd, any amalgam of humans in the same area produces hypnosis. The famous mob mentality is proved that you will act in ways no stage hypnotist could reproduce on stage when they energy of the mob around you – drives you. Pure trance.

Or the army or your group friends – Peer Pressure. As you parents always chided you – "If all your friends jumped off a bridge, would you?" Probably. Your parents would too. Jump off the bridge to fight some distant war that only a politician has a desire for. Buy a certain brand for years because they are the 'best' – without having any idea what goes on in the minds of the people who create that brand, and their concern for stock price increase.

However, you probably want mentioned what is called Brain Washing. The favored 'hypnosis' method of movies and drama. Where changes are created in someone's way of thinking without that person's consent and often against his will. This takes serious time and effort. You require the spirit to be broken and then rebuilt. It is presumed – given enough time and enough resources it can be done to anyone. Not just changing your mind – but changing it against your will.

However, the famous Chinese Brain Washing in the Korean Conflict or Vietnam never changed any American Soldier into a confirmed communist – and torture seemed to work much better in getting what they wanted. So, brain washing is a good story – but possibly that's all.

Our minds are malleable - but our minds are also incredibly powerful. And the more aware we are of the possibilities, and our tendency to making easy quick decisions based on another's suggestion or misdirection – the more self-aware in other words – the more power we have, the more we can use the minds realty to guide our own lives, not lead us on, or let other lead us on in our complacency with damaging beliefs and vague promises.

Our minds are infinitely malleable – that's why NLP works – suggestions directly to and through the conscious mind to changing habits and programs in the subconscious. Sales training is all about working with the conscious mind and its malleability.

Bu this means you too can work on that for your own gain. The renown Hypnotist, Melissa Tiers has several books on how you can use these tools for your own benefit- the most famous one being the "Anti-Anxiety Tool kit"

Hypnosis is a great tool, both for control of others and of yourself.

Be aware of the control that is being exerted – and be aware of the control you can have.

Remember all hypnosis is self-hypnosis.

So we are allowing those others into heads. It may be just the choice of this brand over that – this cereal is better than that (for no apparent reason other than misdirection by advertising – or association from childhood). It may be a vote we wouldn't have made if we had the correct information. Or it may be the whipped-up fear or rage a politician carefully to create.

Be aware. Not scared. Not worried about every action or reaction.

But be aware of your minds process and then become responsible for your actions.

To achieve this use self-hypnosis or meditation or mindfulness or anything to allow you mind to clear and be quite and take stock. A small moment in your life that allows you to reassess what is happening to you.

The media and information networks like to say how bad everything is becoming.

But remember there is an agenda there – bad news sells.

Fear creates calls to action. There are always more people doing good wonderful things in the world than there are bad actions. But the media focus on those with power and those with power tend to want only two things – keep the existing power and get more power.

The rest of the world, mostly cares about their families and their neighbors and are doing untold good, non-newsworthy deeds. Good deeds with no brand or agenda attached. Just because it isn't on the 11 o'clock news doesn't mean it isn't happening –

in abundance.

PART TWO

An examination of Hypnosis and its Possibilities – in dialogue

Imagining Conversations with Ines Simpson.

Mark and Ines discuss and debate Hypnosis

What's wrong with Hypnosis?

MARK: What's wrong with Hypnosis?

INES: I didn't say there way anything wrong with hypnosis.

MARK: You just said I don't like Hypnosis.

INES: The word 'Hypnosis'.

MARK: Same thing.

INES: Couldn't be more different – and how can you say that you being a writer journalist thing and all.

MARK: Wordsmith if you don't mind – okay so what's wrong with THE WORD 'hypnosis'?

INES: Too small.

MARK: You need more letters?

INES: It conveys a meaning too small.

MARK: Hypnosis?

INES: What does it signify to you – I say Hypnosis what do you think?

MARK: Hypnosis? O you know – eyes closed, weird stuff, people slumped in chairs, sleeping but not- the usual.

INES: You see.

MARK: And what does it mean to you?

INES: Doesn't matter what it means to me what it actually is –

MARK: Yes it does.

INES: That's not the point I am on at the moment.

MARK: O excuse me – pray continue with your moment.

SILENCE

MARK Okay - what is it actually then? Hypnosis.

INES: Well...let's say, among other things, it's one of our most direct methods in directly accessing our minds or perhaps The Mind.

MARK: Well okay...people slumped over eyes closed, AND mind stuff.

INES: Yes, except mind stuff as you say its pretty much all there is.

MARK: I don't think -

INES: Tell me something that exists – apart from your mind.

MARK: What? What does that even mean? How -

INES: Alright tell me something that exists for you that doesn't come from what you think or see or perceive or imagine. Or dream.

MARK: Well... There I have picked up a pen, I am holding a pen – without thinking.

INES: But not without perceiving and what part of you perceives that?

MARK: What does that mean I am holding a pen – and you can see that too – so it's an objective ...whatdoyoucall it - objective thingy.

INES: You perceive me through your senses that exist in your brain waves, your touch is a firing of patterns in your brain. You perceive me, the pen, the world, only through senses that are filtered to what you can understand by brain signals.

MARK: Or not

INES: If you think so.

MARK: So you are saying there is nothing existing outside of my head – not you, not the world – not my last bonus cheque –

thank you for that by the way -

INES: O no – I am not saying that.

MARK: I think you are.

INES: You think.

MARK: I...ok so am I wrong?

INES: No way of knowing is there.

MARK: Well, science-

INES: We could say that Science is brain waves studying perceptions

MARK: We could say it was a way of measuring what is True

INES: We could say it was Cornflakes it doesn't make it so

MARK: Alright alright – let's say there is only personal perception.

INES: Ah but there isn't.

MARK: Wow why didn't I think of that –

INES: There is always the mind or minds, wherein all that perception lies.

MARK: Wherein?

INES: Wherein.

MARK: Ok so the mind part, stuff …?

INES: The part that isn't what we direct perceive.

MARK: The unconscious.

INES: Another wobbly word.

MARK: But you know what I mean.

INES: Actually, no .I know what I mean when I say that – but I am never sure of what anyone else says when they say that.

MARK: And that's why we have definitions – to nail down the wobbly bits.

INES: What is the definition of unconscious?

MARK: I don't know right this second – but I could look it up.

INES: You could – but the question here is -what do you mean when you say that word?

MARK: What do you mean?

INES: I asked first.

MARK: Ah you are not sure either –

INES: I know what I mean but I am not sure if I put that knowing into words it will be the same thing. Probably not. Probably less

MARK: That is what one could call a circular argument.

INES: It's not circular – it's wobbly.

MARK: Whatever – so as I understand you, which of course is a wobbly concept - there is what we perceive which is pretty much everything – and then the rest of everything – which is the mind.

INES: And what would you say is a larger – what you know or what you don't know.

MARK: How can we know that?

INES: Exactly.

MARK: Circular.

INES: Which is why I don't like the word hypnosis on most days – too small – especially if it encompasses things that are what we know and don't know.

MARK: Yikes.

INES: Alright. To complete the circular thing if you like —

hypnosis, at its best, is a way, it seems of allowing us to access

the universe of the mind, to get in some measure, outside of

our limited filtered perceptions. In fact to perhaps touch

something infinite for once.

MARK Double Yikes.

INES: Never mind.

MARK: No no, it's good. So hypnosis can touch the infinite. Nice

phrase.

INES: And the problem with things of the mind when you bring

them back into our filters, the brain, our conscious

understanding, they have to fit into limited perceptions.

MARK: Unless like me - you are all powerful because I am clean

of heart and soul, and all understanding.

INES: Yes unless that.

Is Hypnosis real?

Mark: You said if hypnosis is real -Reality is then open to interpretation.

Pause

Mark: You said - Changing truth or -

Ines: I don't think I said that.

Mark: Yes – or it's on your Instagram…or something.

Ines: Hmm… I don't think you quite get the premise behind Instagram.

Mark: So you don't think that?

Ines: That Instagram is a commercial enterprise looking for profit and, not an oracle sent by God?

Mark: Ok that too - but I mean that Hypnosis is an alternate Reality.

Ines: Hypnosis is an altered state perhaps?

Mark: That.

Ines: Yes, I will agrees with that.

Mark: Hypnosis is some form of mind altering -

Ines: No.

Mark: Hypnosis thinks it changes truth or -

Ines: No.

Mark: Ok so - what is hypnosis?

Ines: Open to discussion.

Pause

Mark: Ok let's start again-Is hypnosis real?

Ines: Real? Now you know mostly with the mind, we talk in code words.

Mark: Who does?

Ines: The Mind, Sub-Conscious, Superconscious, levels of hypnosis, ultra-depth, ultra-height on and on – they are not real, but we use the words, because we know from experience the things that happen at these – well let's call them 'levels...or 'places'.'.

Mark: And who knows the code?

Ines: Apparently whatever we connect with when we say 'our mind'.

Mark: And?

Ines: It's a way of conveying intention – we use words, because we have to – though on occasion I have used telepathy.

Mark: No you haven't.

Silence

Mark: Hey!

Mark: Anyway- what I want to know is it real?

Ines: I don't think you grasp the concept of code words.

Mark: Real - you know...ok if I say I have a fear of ...the dark, and the boogeyman. You know I am frightened there are ghosts under my bed and cant sleep - that's not real.

Ines: Which part?

Mark: Well the ghosts under the bed, the boogeyman.

Ines: The fear is real.

Mark: Yes the fear is real - but it's based on...untruth.

Ines: I am not sure truth or untruth are terms that are going to be helpful here. The fear is real.

Mark: So even though it's based on - well bullshit - hypnosis can deal with it - because hypnosis can deal with bullshit.

Ines: Again terms like 'bullshit' and 'truth' are fairly nebulous terms in a discussion unless you clearly define then. Not just now but for all time.

Mark: Define 'truth' - or 'bullshit'? Look you know what I am saying.

Ines: I do.

Mark: What am I saying?

Ines: You want to discuss hard absolutes and then you bring in words like Truth and Real — which in fact are nebulous terms.

Mark: Bullshit.

Ines: Yes sorry and bullshit.

Mark: I mean bullshit — truth and real are hard absolute — true terms.

Ines: Ok.

Mark: Aren't they. I mean what's true is true right?

Ines: Have you heard of the book 'The man who thought his wife was a hat'.

Mark: A cat?

Ines: A hat.

Mark: I don't read fantasy fiction thank you.

Ines: Oliver Sacks wrote it — a doctor — who specialised in brain malfunctions. He wrote among other things this book where the man's brain create the real reality where wherever he looked at his wife he saw a hat.

Mark: An anomaly.

Ines: How about children's reality where there are imaginary friends and animals. And ghosts.

Mark: Those are kids.

Ines: How about when you lose your keys and you search everywhere – and then you look again, in an altered state perhaps and there they are – where you just looked.

Mark: Never happens.

Ines: Or you are looking for a book, and you remember it has a red cover and you search the house and its nowhere, and then your wife says – this book?   And you see it has a grey cover.

Mark: My wife?

Ines: You saw only books with red covers, and couldn't see books with grey covers – you had altered reality.

Mark: I don't get that. Look -A chair is a chair is a chair.

Ines: As a word – not as an absolute.

Mark: But still a chair.

Ines: To you, because -

Mark: To everyone.

Ines: Not to a baby, not to a person who has never seen a chair, in fact if you have never seen furniture and lived say in a jungle all your life – you might not even know where your chair ends and the table begins.

Mark: Oh Bullshit – everyone.

Ines: And possibly not to an alien who sees in 3D.

Mark: No-one sees in 3D- and aliens don't count.

Ines: ooh –Racist!

Mark: The point is. The point is reality is not optional. It is. It always- well IS.

Ines: Hold your hand out - quite stiff - clasp your hands together - now relax and let your imagination work...ok?...now- imagine I am tightening and tightening your hands, as if I am closing a vice over them...tightening and tightening....tighter and tighter forcing them tighter and tighter.

Pause

Mark: Now open your hands. What's the matter?

Ines: Why can't you open your hand?

Mark: I don't know. You -

Ines: Look at me, look at me -Mark you know you can open your hands - open your hands.

Mark: Fuck....and that's a trick.

Ines: Of the mind. It altered your reality.

Mark: No that was a trick.

Ines: Or the time of your heart attack that was indigestion.

Mark: It felt like a heart attack.

Ines: You believed it was.

Mark: It was agony -You called 911 -You believed it too.

Ines: But your body had indigestion - your mind was having a heart attack.

Mark: Whatever - it was painful - it could have been a heart attack.

Ines: It could have been whatever you imagined it to be.

Mark: Ok how about this if there was a court of law -

Ines: O God.

Mark: And a girl was bringing a suit for abuse or rape - and they asked you to hypnotise her and you know bring her back-

Ines: Regress.

Mark: Yes to find out if it was true.

Ines: Again I don't think you quite grasp point of the justice system.

The justice system is about bringing blame - pain to someone. Hypnosis is about removing pain. If this woman or girl truly believed she was abused - she was abused - her body can show the signs even if there was no physical contact. The point is I would want to relive the pain - take away the trauma – if probably not the belief of the event – but take the energy out of the event. The law wants to create pain.

Mark: But what is the truth?

Ines: Indeed.

Mark: Forget it.

Ines: Good idea.

What's Hypnosis got to do with it?

MARK: They say we are either moving to Happiness or to Pain – what's hypnosis ever got to do with that ? Huh!

INES: Are you mad at me for something?

MARK: It's a question. Simple question. With all your talk of consciousness and sub consciousness and mind model bullshit – what that has to do with the real world.

INES: How about this – breathe in

MARK: NO.

INES: Breathe in.

MARK: Is this Hypnosis?

INES: Breathe in...go on.

Pause

INES Good now hold it ...hold it...ok now breathe out.

Pause

MARK: Ok now what?

INES: Repeat.

Pause

MARK My Mom is sick – very sick. Again. And I'm worried.

INES: Ah.

MARK: They don't know what it is.

INES: Who's they?

MARK: The doctors.

INES: Ah.

Pause

MARK: And I was thinking when it gets to be real – like my mother...sick -dying – what's all this Hypnosis we talk about got to do with that?

INES: I guess it has to do with that as much as anything has.

MARK: Look at recent discoveries in medicine. New treatments new process for cancer treatment and Alzheimer's, chronic pain, migraines – what's hypnosis done lately?

INES: What new processes exactly.

MARK: Well there's that study with chronic pain –

INES: And by chronic pain we mean a pain that doctors have no idea of the cause – a mystery but let call it something – we need a name -let's call it... chronic pain – or Bursitis or Crones or- something – because there's an app for that!!

MARK: Bullshit. And now with MRI scans or something they can scan down to the genetic level –

INES: I think you may mean cellular level.

MARK: You see.

INES: And then what do they do?

MARK: I don't know – but then they know stuff – or more stuff.

INES: And then what do they do?

MARK: Stuff. How do I know. I am not a doctor – they give them medicine.

INES: Drugs.

MARK: They do surgery.

INES: So not so much a treatment as a wounding. Not always good to have parts of you hacked off I think.

MARK: If it saves your life? Anyway the thing is what has hypnosis done lately?

INES: You know I do like that you said we are either moving to pain or to – what did you say Happiness? Seems a bit vague – happiness – I would say we are either moving to Love or to Pain.

MARK: Whatever.

INES: Well let's take a 'what if?'

MARK: What if?

INES: What if dis-ease is caused by suppressed or unreleased emotions. Blocked or suppressed thought patterns?

MARK: What – have you heard of viruses by any chance?

INES: What if viruses and let's say bacteria that cause dis-ease are perhaps symptoms not causes.

MARK: Of course they are causes.

INES: Ok and what cause viruses?

MARK: Disease.

INES: Hmm a little circular in your thinking wouldn't you say? And not too helpful in getting rid of the sickness.

MARK: Anger causes cancer is that what you are saying?

INES: Well usually a feeling of rejection or buried unworthiness seems to cause a lot of cancer but you get that idea.

MARK: That's bullshit.

INES: Ok.

MARK: You agree.

INES: No I am trying to move you from pain and anger to – love.

MARK: Fuck you.

INES: And not succeeding.

MARK: Your ridiculous – emotions cause disease! Malaria is cause by mosquitos. Cancer is caused by – rampaging cells – dementia is caused by ...something... lack of iron or fat cells or something – everyone knows that.

INES: It seems, my experience is – in hypnosis -if we release the emotion then the dis-ease seems to go away.

MARK: Bullshit.

INES: Crazy isn't it –

MARK: You mean all these Scan MRI whatever machines and drugs are the wrong way to go – the history of medicine has been a waste of time. Your crazy – we are healthier, we live longer and have cured most crippling diseases - and you say -

INES: Well I would suggest we have taken away most chronic dis-ease and live longer because of clean drinking water, sanitation and possibly penicillin – but that's just me.

MARK: We have almost eradicated breast cancer and... well a whole bunch of stuff. And now they are working on the mental illnesses- that's the next thing.

INES: Is it?

MARK: Anxiety and Distress – according to the US drug companies there are more mental illness and chronic anxieties than ever – specifically mental illness and anxiety. Mental illness is the number one concern of health professionals right now.

INES: Seems to me, perhaps, that dis-ease is taking another course

MARK: What?

INES: Anxiety mental instability is rampant in this healthy society? Look like we have a problem Houston.

MARK: And hypnosis fixes it!

INES: If we take your statement that in this life we are either moving to pain or to Love-

MARK: I said Happiness, happiness – its in the constitution. Pursuit of Happiness

INES: You know the 'pursuit of happiness' was a last minute fudge – they meant prosperity, well being and thriving.

MARK: Same same.

INES: Thriving and well being are so Not - Anxiety and Distress I would say.

MARK: The point is-

INES: The advantage of hypnosis is we can move people more to love and away from pain. And by moving them towards love or well being, if you wish – it doesn't just seem to reduce the pain in their lives – it can, in fact delete it.

MARK: So hypnosis cures people.

INES: I am saying we move people towards thriving and well being – and away from strife and anxiety.

MARK: And you don't think that what is medicine is doing?

INES: Rampant plagues of mental illness would seem to answer that question.

MARK: Its not that there are more, or its new - its that we can label them now.

INES: Ah labels – so popular with the drug companies and the DSM.

MARK: What's the DSN?

INES: DSM - Look it up. Listen I am not saying that doctors don't want to help.

MARK: Fucking doctors.

PAUSE

INES: I am sorry about your mother.

Pause

MARK: Maybe you could see her?

INES : Does she want me to see her?

MARK: She's never heard of you.

INES: Yes you see Hypnosis is about an agreement and willingness to create change – your own change. Its not the last possible option miracle crazy drug you take or force on someone -hoping and trying and desperate.

MARK: So – what I should talk to her?...Maybe I'll talk to her.

INES: And say what?

MARK: That you will help her with her sickness?

INES: Her sickness? I though you said she was ill – is she making the sickness a personal thing ?

MARK No – you know what I mean – its just a ...thing.. a way of saying...

INES: Thinking.

MARK So I shouldn't talk to her – she should just suffer?

INES: If she is willing to get well, and she is willing to opt for change – then sure I will talk to her.

MARK: Of course she is willing to get well.

INES: Ok.

MARK: You think she isn't?

INES: I have no idea – but hypnosis isn't surgery where we cut off bits and then hope. Its an approach to change. It involves a willingness to change.

MARK: Whatever.

Pause

MARK: I'll talk to her.

If Hypnosis was a thing – it would be taught in Medical school

MARK: If Hypnosis was a thing it would be taught in medical school.

INES: You could say- if Life was a thing it would be taught in medical school – but mostly it's about symptoms and illness.

MARK: Low blow.

INES: You know who developed modern hypnosis?

MARK: The amazing Kerskin?

INES: So close. All modern hypnosis ideas and training come from the medical profession. Dr Esdaile, Dr James Braid, Dr Bettleheim, neurologist Jean-Martin Charcot,Dr Erickson, etc. etc

MARK: Yea? So who's that radio guy you like – he wasn't a doctor.

INES: Radio guy?

MARK: Played trumpet or something.

INES: Dave Elman?

MARK: Yea Dave Elman band – and that other trickster – Kein.

INES: Gerald Kein – teacher and learned -

MARK: Yea that's it Jerry Kein – stage Hypnotist -and Elman radio announcer - how close did those two ever get to medical school?

INES: I'm sure they passed a couple on their way to work.

MARK: You know if Hypnosis was any good it would be prescribed.

INES: Now there's a stunning definition of what's good. Prescribed like thalidomide perhaps?

MARK: That's –

INES: Or perhaps -Norodin- or let's call it Methamphetamine or Quaaludes or Morphine or Pentobarbital   - all good drugs –now known killers-

MARK: The point is –

INES: I know if God had wanted us to have Hypnosis – he would have made it a natural thing...Oh wait – it is!

MARK: No it isn't.

INES: Define Hypnosis.

MARK: When you go gaga and bark like a chicken and click like a dog.

INES: Yep – you've almost got it.

MARK: Am I wrong?

INES: Hypnosis is what happens when your mind changes its state and become focused – such as when you watch a movie or read a book. If there wasn't hypnosis there would be no suspension of disbelief – or as we professionals like to say – by pass of the critical factor. If Hypnosis wasn't natural we would just end up in a theatre watching light and color. Reading a book would be a bunch of words at random on a page. Imagination is Hypnosis. Being 'in the zone' is Hypnosis. Being in a state of fear is Hypnosis. Being in Lust is in Hypnosis .When you go to Hospital you go -

MARK:I don't think that's Hypnosis.

PAUSE

INES: Well...

MARK: Well it's just my opinion.

INES: Always good to have opinions.

MARK: I'm entitled to my opinions am I not?

INES: Long as it doesn't interfere with reality or anything else vaguely important.

MARK: Right. Exactly.

INES Or talking to me.

MARK: What?

MARK: Hey. Hey now where are you going...

What's the deal with Fields?

MARK: So what's this about fields?

INES: Fields? Fields as in flowers?

MARK: No fields as in Quantum.

INES: Ah.

MARK: Yes -what's that about?

INES: I think you might have to narrow the question –
otherwise we might be talking about infinity. Or flowers.

MARK: Well you're always talking about it. Fields this field that.
Field theory field – everything.

INES: I do?

MARK: Sure all the time – in Conferences, on the websites –
everywhere.

INES: I do?

MARK: Ok not all the time – but you have mentioned it.

INES: Ah… So what's your question about this field I may have once mentioned?

MARK: Well what is it – I mean what does it do ? In fact whey are you even mentioning it. Quantum. You're a hypnotist.

INES: Female hypnotist.

MARK: I rest my case.

PAUSE

MARK: I was joking.

PAUSE

MARK: Alright alright - I retract and repent. Ok? - I apologise.

PAUSE

INES: May I just say groveling would certainly become you.

MARK: Whatever – so- fields - fields of knowledge – fields of quantum – what?

INES: I think its Morphic fields we are aiming for.

MARK: Not quantum? Everybody says quantum.

INES: We can start with quantum.

MARK: Ok.

INES: It seems – and I say 'its seems', because that what it appears to seem – it seems that there is some web out there- or everywhere in fact.

MARK: Web like spider or web like World Wide Web?

INES Like World Wide – Internet yes –but not limited to – well anything – bigger than worldwide that's for sure. Some connected web of everything that some of us or some part of everything taps into.

Mark: Is there porn on this web too?

INES: For instance we know – when a new idea comes along – an invention – a new way of thinking –

MARK: Like the world is round- not flat.

INES: Mark no-one ever thought the world was flat.

MARK: Columbus was the first guy-

INES: Mark – don't go with what you read on the back of a cornflakes box when you were five – check the information. The ancients knew the world was round. The world looks round – to anyone.

MARK: Those old maps are flat.

INES: Yes – hard to put a globe in a book. What do our maps look like?

MARK: I thought –

INES: Anyway about fields.

PAUSE

INES: Are you pouting now?

MARK: No.

PAUSE

Mark: So continue.

INES: When a new idea comes along – a new way of thinking - an invention – like the steam engine, the telephone, the electric light –even though we are taught in school the BIG MAN THEORY –the special' brilliant but eccentric inventor – in fact historically we know these new ideas suddenly seem to appear in hundreds of places at once – Just because say Edison bullies his way into the History books - doesn't mean he was the sole keeper of that new idea – The electric light, the telephone, the steam engine, the television, the computer were suddenly ideas appearing all across the written world in the same space of time.

We like to have hero narratives so it's always the one GUY – and occasionally, very occasionally the one woman who gets the credit. But because it's written - doesn't make it so.

MARK History is bunk.

INES: No Written history is bunk, and self-congratulatory. But actual History is History. It's just we so love the narrative.

MARK: The back of Cornflake boxes leads the news.

INES: There was the case of birds in England start to peck at the gold seals on milk bottles that were delivered to doorsteps. Because a gold seal meant cream at the top of the bottle. And it happened all across the country when the gold seal bottles came out. Various bottle caps were tried over a number of years but most proved to be ineffective, groups of birds actually waiting for milkmen when they would arrive to make their deliveries each morning, and the behavior spread throughout the European continent.

MARK I heard that.

INES: Or more crazy a new form of crystal is developed in a lab – and within a few weeks that new form of crystal appears in labs all over the western world –as if the new idea had spread among the molecules.

MARK: Ok that's bullshit – pyramids and crystals.

INES: Quantum or more precisely Morphic.

MARK: Meaning?

INES : Fields vibrating and interacting with each other.

MARK: OK so anyway – the fields are...what?

INES: Well in physics they say quantum fields are where the particles – stuff – or waves –that we experience as physical stuff come from. Remember the wave-particle duality?

MARK: No.

INES: Well, you might as well forget about it. In fact, there are no particles and no waves; just fields. Both "particles" and "waves" are merely two ways in which we interpret the physical from quantum fields. To the best of our present 'scientific' ability to perceive and to reason, the universe is made from fields and nothing else, and these fields are not made from any smaller components.

MARK: So basically everything is energy.

INES: So basically everything is connected.

MARK: So basically there is no individual stuff – it's all connected. New age bullshit.

INES: And then of course there is the Morphic field – so called.

MARK OF course – so called. And what then is this field – a different field, from the complete field that is all fields?

INES: I detect sarcasm and skepticism- but as usual, I choose to ignore it.

MARK: Again - Morphic Field ?

INES : Sort of says that all things are fields, within fields.

MARK: Of course it does.

INES: For instance memory is not solely local – there is collective memory – wisdom is not your or mine there seems to be a collective wisdom. And when new knowledge is found it spreads – through the field, or fields, or whatever it is, and so it accessible to all. Fields of memory, fields of knowledge, fields of pain and trauma.

MARK: Nice.

INES: The human condition – trauma and pain.

MARK: Nice. Comforting.

INES: But also there is –

MARK: For the sake of discussion and journalistic balance – let's say – let's just say then that we are immersed in this crap - and so what does that have to do with hypnosis?

INES: For one thing - it seems in Hypnosis, deep states of Hypnosis we have access to these fields - sometimes complete access.

MARK: So?

INES: As a simple example, it is possible to find memories, and events that have caused harm, or trauma, as they are always there - and take away that energy – and so, as far as the Mind is concerned, take away the power of that event.

PAUSE

INES: Of course that is just scratching the surface of the possible – think about it– Hypnosis is about the mind – and the mind floats in these fields, perhaps exists only in these fields - so if we want to-

MARK: Perhaps the mind is a field.

INES: By George - I think he's got it.

MARK: Whatever.

INES: Now repeat after me again – the rain in Spain falls -

MARK: You know - My Fair Lady is perhaps your era – but not mine – the sarcasm will be lost.

INES: Your loss.

MARK: Anyway you know if there was such a thing as this all knowing field -NASA or Homeland Security or all those other secret agencies we know nothing about would have nailed it shut by now – taken everything and then nailed it shut.

INES: We are not separate from – but immersed in. It would be like a fish trying to steal the sea. Where would she put it?

MARK: OK so in Hypnosis you can access these fields – all these fields.

INES: So it seems.

MARK: I can?

INES: You can, he she or it can. The mind does yes.

PAUSE

MARK: Ok so dial me in. I want in. To the knowledge bit – I have enough pain and trauma already. Dial me in to the wisdom bit. Tap in. Think about it - I could learn to play the guitar - 4 languages –cool dance moves -if it creates physical bits – could I have better hair? Does it do the future?

INES: Just because wisdom exists - and is accessible doesn't mean we get it.

MARK: I get it...let's say I get it.

INES: We seem to be only able to embrace and manifest what we are able to accept -

MARK: When the pupil is ready the gold arrives.

INES: Something like that.

MARK: How do we get ready .So how do I do it?

INES: Well that is sort of the eternal question isn't it?

Wrong about Everything

MARK: what if you are wrong?

INES: About what?

MARK: Everything.

INES: Now that is a thought I revisit often.

MARK Right - so how are you sure you are doing the right thing?

INES: I am never sure.

MARK: I mean when you are using hypnosis – maybe you are taking the person in the wrong direction – maybe you are creating some form of harm by working in their mind.

INES: I doubt it.

MARK: Oh so now you are sure.

INES: I am never sure – but as long as I let the client's mind do the work and not my mind, not my judgement not my pre-conditioning then its good - it's the clients mind that does all the work. Not me.

MARK: The client's mind? That's the one that's screwed up. That is why they come to you – no?

INES: Well perhaps not screwed up – but let's say in some form of disarray yes.

MARK: And that's what you trust to do the work?

INES: Well in general in Hypnosis you are working with the subconscious – where the disarray certainly lies – usually – but then it's merely a matter of uncovering the 'sore spot' and allowing self healing.

MARK: They heal themselves.

INES: Who else is going to do it?

MARK: You -the hypnotist! Like a doctor does or a dentist does.

INES: A doctor heals a broken bone?

MARK: Well I mean.

INES: A doctor heals cancer?

MARK : In fact in that case yes.

INES: How?

MARK: I don't know – drugs, chemo – stuff- you know.

INES: Well - I would say the drugs , the chemo, the stuff are merely tools – often invasive I might say – that help or encourage or allow the body to do what it always does – which is heal. We are self healing mechanisms – when given the right environment.

MARK: Yes but –

INES: In Hypnosis the tool is the mind itself – and we- merely the guides – the facilitator – the encouragers if you will.

MARK: Well I think-

INES: Now in the type of Hypnosis I use I tend to by pass even the subconscious and work with the Higher mind of the client – and the Higher mind of the client only has one goal, I find, the best outcome for their host.

MARK: Huh. So the client heals themselves.

INES: Yes.

MARK: So why do we need you – why don't we just heal ourselves?

INES: I know – why can't we?

MARK: I just said that.

INES: Lots of reasons. Mostly because we don't know we can.

MARK: So you must have no problems – you must be a self healed machine.

INES: Me? I'm a mass of walking problems – like anyone.

MARK: I rest my case.

INES: Because I have an ego, I have opinions, I have fears and I have misunderstandings I have doubt.

MARK: Ok – so-

INES: As do all my , or any . client – so my job is   to by pass the ego, uncover the fears and show them to be unneeded, clear the doubt -

MARK: All fears are unneeded? Some fears are healthy otherwise we would be jumping into lions dens willy nilly.

INES: Willy Nilly?

MARK: You know what I mean.

INES: Yes you are right - Sorry I should have said uncover and expose the fears that have no practical purpose in helping the client.

MARK: Ah ! And how do you decide that.

INS: I ask their higher mind to decide that – not my job.

MARK: Here you go again with these wishy washy words – 'Higher mind'.

INES: Wishy Washy – is that like Peely Wally?

MARK: What? Look I like science – facts proofs – where is this 'higher mind'?

INES: I have no idea – is that important to know?

MARK: Of course – we have to know – we have to rest everything on FACT.

INES: Well yes nice to think so.

MARK: Its vital – crucial – its how we function.

INES OK well lets start with a basic fact: -how do you know you exist?

MARK: Because…

INES How do you know you are not a figment of my thought process?

MARK: Not possible – I can prove I exist.

INES: Go ahead.

MARK... well...if I hit you you'll feel it.

INES: And that's proves what? How do you know that's not everything in my head?

MARK: Because I am me.

INES: So you think – maybe I am making you think that?

MATRK No way – ah your driving me crazy.

INES: Maybe that's my plan.

MARK: What ! No! - is it?

INES: Maybe I am a figment of your thought process.

MARK No...no...

INES: How do you know?

MARK Because ...its...

INES: What would it look like if I were - or you were - a figment in my mind.

PAUSE

INES: So now we are not even sure we exist – then as Bertram Russell says – let's just assume we exist for the purpose of this experiment.

MARK: What experiment?

INES: Life.

PAUSE

MARK The point is - I think this past life stuff is bullshit.

INES: O that's the point?

MARK: Really I mean I think its just some justification for hypnotists to make money – have sessions, encourage hallucinations all that.

INES: What if we said it wasn't a separate past life – but a reflection of our journey through the multi universe.

PAUSE

INES You know the 'Scientific' ' Factual' 'Pragmatic' 'Multi Universe' theory right?

MARK: Yes yes.

PAUSE

INES: So there you – multi dimensions of one life...

MARK Okay...okay - I could see that. Different angles of ourselves – in the different possible universes – and...wow yea I see that's possible.

INES: Sure – why not.

MARK: That's what past lives are? None of this malarkey about reincarnation – but really just the different possibilities popping up from all the possible universes

INES: Sure.

MARK: Really?

PAUSE

MARK: But that's not what you think.

INES: Doesn't matter what I think. Its what works.

MARK: You think there really are past lives don't you?

INES: Again it doesn't matter – it's a matter of getting the outcome for the client in the chair. If they are really going to a 'past life' and by going there – in their mind- somehow takes away their anxiety or phobia or physical ailment, or whatever. If it's a multi universe – or merely a metaphor the client's mind uses to get to the problem or ailment- it doesn't matter. We don't need facts – we need paths that get us outcomes.

MARK: See - you do believe there are past lives.

INES: I am merely a figment of your mind – so maybe its you who believe I believe in past lives.

PAUSE

MARK: I hate you .

On Being Analytical

MARK: The point is I am an analytical thinker.

INES: Mark, leave me alone - I am playing Solitaire- and I am happy.

MARK: That's why Hypnosis doesn't make sense to me.

Pause

MARK: You see?

INES: Ok - you know those 2 statements ' I am an analytical thinker 'and 'that's why hypnosis doesn't make sense " -analytically don't make sense.

MARK: Sure it does.

INES: I hate to do this because I was having a nice afternoon -but let me ask – analytical thinking means what exactly – to you?

MARK: You know – I analyse stuff.

INES: Uh huh.

MARK: You know break it down see where the hard facts are.

INES: Uh huh.

MARK: Right?

INES: And which hard facts are we using at this time to 'analyse' hypnosis exactly?

MARK: Well...here's the thing this 'Soul level' and all that – that's definitely bullshit.

INES: Bullshit analytically speaking you mean?

MARK: Yes.

INES: Analytically - bullshit is an emotional response to something that bothers you – emotionally.

MARK: Bullshit.

INES: Has it ever occurred to you that where the 'humans are like analytical computers' analogy is there is no emotional component. And humans are bound up with emotions.

MARK: Says you.

INES: Consider -the theory that we make decisions based on hard facts stuff -is factually and analytically - well - crazy.

MARK: Says you.

INES: We have never – you have never -I have never- humankind has never ever, ever made a step or any decision without a huge emotional involvement in that step.

MARK: You are saying our History is the result of a bunch of nammby pamby- hand wringing cry baby decisions.

INES: Interesting language.

MARK: Bullshit.

INES: Uh huh.

MARK: So ...so Napoleon and Hitler and all the American Leadership and...and - and the fucking N. Koreans all they ever do – all their decisions were just a result of some emotional – bullshit!

INES: You think they aren't?

MARK: We need to think logically

INES: Logically it may be a good idea for us to start thinking logically – but we are emotional beings and therefore incapable of making any decision or having any thought that does not have a large emotional component.

Pause

MARK: You know, I don't even know what that means.

INES: Never mind – can I go back to my Solitaire App now?

Pause

MARK: The thing is...

Pause

MARK: The thing is if you hypnotise me I'm frightened I may do something stupid – or tell you something...or something , or something ...might happen.

Pause

MARK: Will something happen?

INES: What do you think?

MARK: What if I don't want something to happen?

Pause

MARK: Will it help me?

Pause

MARK: I don't need help...really...so...

Pause

MARK: Ok so if I give it a try...

Pause

MARK: What do you think?

Pause

MARK: Are you hypnotizing me now?

Pause

MARK: The thing is...I guess... I trust you- so...

Pause

INES: So shall we begin?

MARK: You tricked me – you manipulated me. Right? This was a set up.

Pause

MARK: Ok do I need an appointment then or...or what?

INES: Do you want to go into hypnosis then. Now?

MARK: I guess.

INES: Not good enough.

MARK: Why?

INES: All hypnosis is self hypnosis – you move yourself into a hypnotic state – I am just the caretaker of the states.

MARK: Sure...what does that mean?

INES: You have Free will. A choice, Always

MARK: So I get to choose.

INES: You always get to choose.

MARK: Fuck!

INES: I know

Hypnosis corrupts

MARK: Hypnosis corrupts people you know.

INES: Indeed? And where does this wonderful revelation come from?

MARK: It's true.

INES: Facebook?.

MARK: YouTube actually.

INES: Oh yes that's even better – cos its video.

MARK: So you agree.

INES: With?

MARK: Hypnosis makes you do things you would never normally do.

INES: Like forgiveness?

MARK: Sex stuff.

INES: O... sex stuff. Is this leading to some sort of personal Las Vegas confession?

MARK : What! No. But Its true.

INES: YouTube.

MARK: Not just YouTube.

INES: Twitter.

MARK: No I mean – haven't you seen those shows – like Vegas stuff.? Sex Hypnosis. On stage.

INES: Surprisingly – No.

MARK: They exist – Vegas sleaze hypnosis stuff.

INES: Oh I am aware . So let me just clarify – do you feel people only do sexual things when hypnotised?

MARK: It's like when you're drunk.

INES: So sex only if drunk or hypnotised.

MARK: No – but the stuff they do.

INES: Ok so people only do weird stuff when drunk or hypnotised.

MARK: Yes.

INES: So this is a personal history thing.

MARK: No – The thing is you guys -

INES: You guys?

MARK: Hypnotists always say – 'now don't worry – you won't do anything you don't want to do – you won't tell me anything you don't want to tell me' – then you zap them - and all kinds of stuff is – well exposed.

INES: Zap?

MARK: You know.

INES : And you have evidence of this then - apart from ..on Twitter?

MARK: It could happen - right?

PAUSE

MARK: Ok I don't know - but what I am saying -

INES: Are you saying that people are morally pure and correct in all things – unless they drink or turn to hypnosis - which is when they morph into monsters?

MARK: Ok maybe not Monsters – exactly. But they do stuff they not would normally do.

INES: Yes again I give you -forgiveness

MARK: No - bad stuff

INES: Oks so let's just say people, on the surface are not the whole thing. In fact I would say under the right circumstance we are pretty much capable of anything – good or bad. Any of us. All of us.

MARK: You agree.

INES: But, strangely, I am not trying to enable my clients to do horrible things. In fact it's to stop the horrible things they usually come to me in the first place.

MARK: But you could.

INES: I could jump in front of a bus – but I won't.

MARK: But others could – that's my point.

INES: If your point is that if a person wanted to corrupt another or others, and they were determined and dedicated – they could do it. Well welcome to the real world of 2017.

MARK: You see – it's a terrible thing.

INES: I agree – though to blame Hypnosis is like blaming breathing.

MARK: No because –

INES: Hypnosis is a part of how we are – its when we change a state – and like every other part of us – it goes where we go. I happen to use it to help people. But if you just want to make money and bend people to your way of thinking – how far do you have to look? The Media, Government, Advertising, Corporations, Big Pharma, Big -

MARK: Yea - So what's the answer?

INES: What's the question?

MARK: How do we – protect ourselves from things like that?

INES: Advertising?

MARK: Hypnosis? All of it.

INES: Protect ourselves? From Hypnosis? You know I really don't think there is, currently anyway, an epidemic of fatal hypnosis events caused by hypnotists .

Pause

MARK: So you think Hypnotism is a good thing?

INES: I do.

MARK: Despite all we have just said.

INES: Let me expose to you a little known Hypnosis secret...Ok?

MARK: Sure - yeah - tell me.

INES: To make someone do something that's a radical 360 from their everyday lives takes a lot of work. I am talking sleep deprivation, time manipulation, solitary confinement, ideally where no-one can hear them yelling, constant interrogations, ideally some torture – possibly a lot of torture. And then time - maybe 3 months, 6 months - a year. A lot of constant work, dedication and attention to details – and then, even then there's no guarantee...

MARK: Yes but -

INES: And you know - that is hard to achieve in a one or two hour session in a comfortable recliner in my office.

MARK: The thing is -

INES: Just to convince someone to buy a certain brand of Soap takes millions of dollars spent on time and effort - and constant repetition over months. Years. Just to buy Soap. But it can be done . I give you Proctor and Gamble.

PAUSE

MARK: So there is no answer...to the question -is what you are saying?

INES: The question being ... 'how do we protect ourselves from ourselves' ?

MARK: Yes - exactly.

INES: I think the answer is in the question.

Pause

MARK: No it's not – hey where are you going – we haven't finished this – that's not an answer – is that answer ?

MARK: Hey!

Who is Ines Simpson?

Ines Simpson – a bio

Ines has worked in many fields from the hospitality industry to commercial fishing on Canada's west coast. In her 40's, she started to reevaluate her life and to search for something that would fulfill her and give her life more meaning. Finally, in the late 90s her mother (!) took a hypnotherapy course and a light bulb went on! The rest as they say is history!

However as you don't know the history –we will tell it- but we will be brief.

Ines became a member of the National Guild of Hypnotists in 2000 - the National Guild is the largest hypnosis body in the world. By 2005, she was admitted as a faculty member   and then as a Board Certified Hypnotist making her the first certified instructor for the NGH in western Canada. She was inducted in 2012 to the NGH's Order of Braid in recognition of service to professional hypnotism. She also searched out Gerald Kein and was taught and mentored by him to become one of the very few DCI Certified Omni Hypnosis

Instructors in N America – Omni is one the most respected Hypnosis Trainings in the world.

Ines Simpson along the way, in an effort to both simplify and deepen her Hypnotist Practice, and more importantly to effect the best outcomes for her clients, developed a system that has become known as the Simpson Protocol.

The Simpson Protocol, is the only way known today to effectively communicate with hypnosis clients in the Esdaile State and beyond.   For the first time, the hypnotist can converse with the client's deepest mind to learn what the true issues are and to direct it to do what is needed to achieve the best results possible. The Protocol also allows the Hypnotist to effect huge outcomes without ever having to know the particulars of the issues involved. It seems the Hypnotist's ego is taken out of the equation, and the most powerful and knowing force in the room (for the Client)- the Clients Mind - does all the work.

The Esdaile State is also the launching pad into higher and deeper states of hypnosis, which is allowing The Simpson Protocol Students and Practitioners to expand and develop the system in ,it seems, unlimited directions.

"Ines Simpson is a very respected hypnotist and lecturer on the Esdaile State. [S]he is widely regarded as one of the top experts in the world. I came away impressed with her professional expertise, but also with her character. She never hesitates to say "I don't know" or "Not proven yet." And THAT level of humility and honesty is not always present in world-class experts."
– H. Larry Elman (Dave Elman's son)

"*I have worked with Ines Simpson as the Simpson Protocol evolved and often co-present with her during live teaching sessions. She is brilliant, yet humble and unassuming. She loves to teach and impart what she knows to others. I have personally worked with her as a client and have had some amazing results using her protocol. I highly recommend her to anyone who really wants to make changes in their life."*

-TED ROBINSON – center for Inner Healing

"Ines, I just wanted to say how outstanding your one-day training session on working in the Esdaile state and beyond was last weekend. It really opened my eyes about an entirely new aspect of hypnosis/hypnotherapy and working with people in those deep states and the results you can get. Plus you were so kind and compassionate with those of us undergoing the experience as well as being trained in using it.   The whole thing was really mind expanding – dare I say mind blowing – and I want to thank you again for the fabulous job you did in taking us to new depths – and heights.   Looking forward to more training with you in the near future, Ines."

Mike Hulme, BA,DC,CHT

" I am very fortunate to live in an area of the world that has a hypnotherapist instructor of Ines Simpson`s caliber. I am still awed at the depth of her commitment to furthering the profession of Hypnotherapy"

Dave Bartlett, Campbell River, British Columbia

LINKS

Ines Simpson Website and info

https://inessimpson.com

For Self Hypnosis on-line:

http://selfhypnosis.esdaileinstitute.com/

For an Introduction to Hypnosis:

Free Video Series for Hypnosis

Hypnosis Training and Information:

https://esdaileinstitute.com/

Advanced Hypnosis Info & Training :

https://simpsonprotocol.com/

'Hypnosis-Everywhere' – The Podcast/Radio show

http://hypnosis.simpsonprotocol.com/

Printed by: SimpsonProtocol press
Copyright © 2018 inessimpson.com

For more information on this or other ines simpson publications
Contact me at ines@inessimpson.com,